THE MOST PROVEN AND EFFECTIVE WAY TO ACHIEVE WEIGHT LOSS

A Comprehensive Guide to Mastering Weight Loss, Eat Less, Exercise, and Achieve Balance for Healthy and Sustainable Weight Management

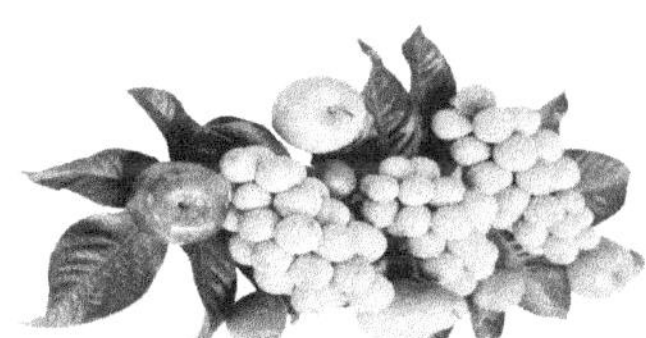 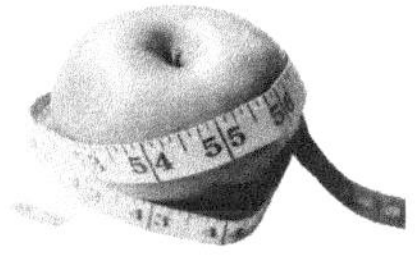

Joyce M. Baker

All rights reserved. No part of this publication may be reproduced, distributed, or transmitted in any form or by any means, including photocopying, recording, or other electronic or mechanical methods, without the prior written permission of the publisher, except in the case of brief quotations embodied in critical reviews and certain other non commercial uses permitted by the copyright law.

ABOUT THE AUTHOR

The author of "The Most Proven and Effective Way to Achieve Weight Loss" is Joyce M. Baker, a renowned nutritionist and fitness expert with over 15 years of experience in the field. Joyce holds a PhD in Nutritional Sciences and is dedicated to promoting evidence-based approaches to weight management. Her passion for helping individuals achieve their health goals shines through in her comprehensive understanding of nutrition, exercise physiology, and behavior change strategies. Through her writing and consulting, Joyce M. Baker has empowered countless people to take control of their health and transform their lives.

TABLE OF CONTENT

INTRODUCTION

Overview of the book's purpose and the importance of achieving weight loss in a healthy manner.
Achieving weight loss involves a combination of healthy eating, regular physical activity, and lifestyle changes.

Overview:
"The Most Proven and Effective Way to Achieve Weight Loss" is a comprehensive guidebook designed to educate and empower individuals seeking to achieve weight loss in a healthy and sustainable manner. Authored by renowned nutrition and fitness experts, this book provides readers with evidence-based strategies, practical tips, and motivational insights to support them on their weight loss journey.

Purpose:

The primary purpose of "The Most Proven and Effective Way to Achieve Weight Loss" is to address the widespread issue of obesity and overweight while offering a solution-oriented approach to weight management. Recognizing the numerous challenges individuals face in their quest for weight loss, the book aims to provide clear guidance on adopting healthy lifestyle habits that promote long-term success. By dispelling myths, providing accurate information, and offering actionable advice, the book empowers readers to take control of their health and achieve their weight loss goals effectively.

Importance of Achieving Weight Loss in a Healthy Manner:

The book emphasizes the importance of achieving weight loss in a healthy manner for several key reasons:

- *Long-Term Health:* Rapid or unsustainable weight loss methods can have detrimental effects on overall health, including nutrient deficiencies, muscle loss, and metabolic disruptions. By promoting healthy weight loss strategies, the book prioritizes long-term health and well-being.

- *Sustainable Results:* Crash diets and extreme weight loss measures often result in short-term success followed by rapid weight regain. In contrast, adopting healthy lifestyle habits, such as balanced nutrition and regular exercise, fosters sustainable weight loss that can be maintained over time.

- *Prevention of Chronic Diseases:* Obesity is a significant risk factor for various chronic diseases, including heart disease, type 2 diabetes, and certain cancers. By achieving weight loss through healthy means, individuals can reduce their risk of developing these serious health conditions and improve their overall quality of life.

- *Positive Body Image:* Focusing solely on the number on the scale can lead to negative body image and self-esteem issues. "The Best Way to Achieve Weight Loss" encourages readers to adopt a holistic approach to health and wellness, promoting self-acceptance, body positivity, and self-care practices.

- *Behavioral Changes:* Healthy weight loss involves not only physical changes but also behavioral and psychological shifts. The book addresses the importance of mindset, self-awareness, and goal-setting in facilitating lasting behavior change, empowering readers to overcome obstacles and maintain healthy habits for life.

Overall, "The Most Proven and Effective Way to Achieve Weight Loss" serves as a valuable resource for anyone seeking practical guidance and inspiration to embark on a journey towards improved health, vitality, and self-confidence through sustainable weight management practices.

Brief discussion on the prevalence of obesity and its impact on health.

Obesity is a growing global health concern with significant implications for individual health and well-being, as well as public health systems. The prevalence of obesity has reached epidemic proportions worldwide, affecting people of all ages, genders, socioeconomic backgrounds, and ethnicities.

Statistics reveal alarming trends in obesity rates over the past few decades. According to the World Health Organization (WHO), global obesity rates have nearly tripled since 1975. In 2016, more than 1.9 billion adults were overweight, and of these, over 650 million were obese. Additionally, the prevalence of childhood obesity has increased dramatically, with the number of overweight or obese children under the age of five estimated to be over 40 million globally.

The impact of obesity on health is profound and multifaceted, affecting virtually every organ system in the body. Some of the key health consequences of obesity include:

- *Cardiovascular Disease:* Obesity is a major risk factor for heart disease, including hypertension, coronary artery disease, stroke, and heart failure. Excess body fat can lead to elevated blood pressure, abnormal lipid levels, and inflammation, all of which contribute to cardiovascular dysfunction.

- *Type 2 Diabetes:* Obesity is strongly associated with the development of type 2 diabetes, a metabolic disorder characterized by insulin resistance and high blood sugar levels. The accumulation of visceral fat, particularly around the abdomen, disrupts insulin signaling pathways and impairs glucose regulation.

- *Cancer:* Obesity has been linked to an increased risk of various types of cancer, including breast, colorectal, endometrial, kidney, pancreatic, and liver cancer. Adipose tissue produces hormones and inflammatory substances that promote tumor growth and metastasis.

- *Respiratory Disorders:* Obesity can adversely affect lung function and increase the risk of respiratory conditions such as obstructive sleep apnea, asthma, and obesity hypoventilation syndrome. Excess weight puts pressure on the chest wall and diaphragm, leading to breathing difficulties.

- *Musculoskeletal Issues:* The additional weight carried by obese individuals puts strain on the musculoskeletal system, leading to joint pain, osteoarthritis, and mobility limitations. Obesity-related joint stress can accelerate cartilage degeneration and exacerbate existing orthopedic problems.

- *Mental Health Disorders:* Obesity is associated with an increased risk of depression, anxiety, low self-esteem, and body image dissatisfaction. Psychosocial factors, societal stigma, and discrimination against individuals with obesity can further exacerbate mental health issues.

- *Gastrointestinal Disorders:* Obesity is linked to a higher prevalence of gastrointestinal conditions such as gastroesophageal reflux disease (GERD), fatty liver disease, gallstones, and certain digestive cancers.

The economic burden of obesity on healthcare systems is substantial, encompassing direct medical costs, productivity losses, and decreased quality of life. Addressing the prevalence of obesity requires a comprehensive, multi-sectoral approach that encompasses public health initiatives, policy changes, community interventions, and individual behavior modification strategies. By raising awareness of the health risks associated with obesity and promoting preventive measures, we can work towards reducing its impact on both individual and population health.

CHAPTER 1: UNDERSTANDING WEIGHT LOSS

Explanation of the basic principles of weight loss, including calorie deficit and metabolism.

Understanding the basic principles of weight loss is essential for anyone seeking to achieve and maintain a healthy body weight.

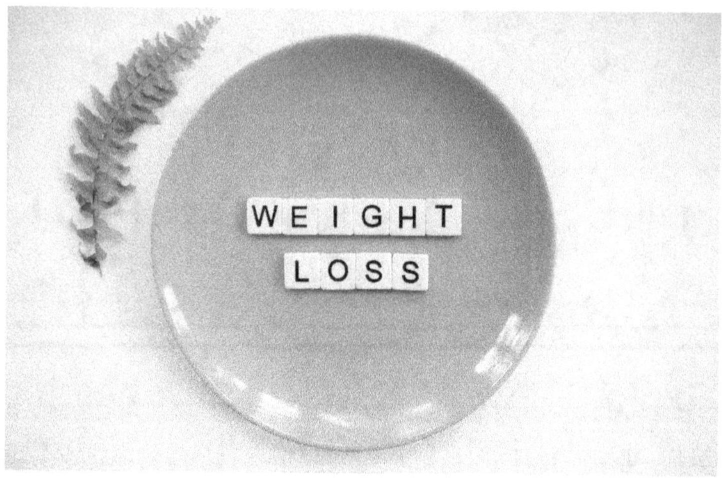

Two fundamental concepts at the core of weight loss are calorie deficit and metabolism.

1. Calorie Deficit:

A calorie deficit occurs when you consume fewer calories than your body expends over a given period.

To lose weight, you must create a calorie deficit, meaning you need to burn more calories than you consume.

This deficit can be achieved through a combination of reducing calorie intake (diet) and increasing calorie expenditure (physical activity).

One pound of body weight is roughly equivalent to 3,500 calories. Therefore, to lose one pound per week, you would need to create a calorie deficit of approximately 500 calories per day.

It's important to create a moderate calorie deficit that allows for steady, sustainable weight loss without compromising nutrient intake or metabolic rate.

2. Metabolism:

Metabolism refers to the processes by which your body converts food and drink into energy to sustain life and perform various bodily functions.

Basal metabolic rate (BMR) is the number of calories your body needs to maintain basic physiological functions while at rest.

Factors influencing metabolism include age, gender, body composition, genetics, and hormonal status.

Muscle mass plays a significant role in metabolism, as muscle tissue burns more calories at rest compared to fat tissue.

Physical activity and exercise also impact metabolism, as they increase energy expenditure and can elevate metabolic rate both during and after activity.

Certain dietary factors, such as the thermic effect of food (TEF), also influence metabolism. Protein has a higher thermic effect compared to carbohydrates and fats, meaning it requires more energy to digest and metabolize.

Adequate hydration is important for maintaining optimal metabolic function, as dehydration can negatively impact metabolic rate.

While metabolism varies from person to person, there are strategies to support a healthy metabolism, including regular physical activity, strength training to build muscle mass, consuming a balanced diet rich in whole foods, and getting sufficient sleep.

Weight loss occurs when you create a calorie deficit through a combination of reduced calorie intake and increased calorie expenditure. Understanding and implementing these basic principles, along with adopting healthy lifestyle habits, can support successful and sustainable weight loss efforts. Additionally, supporting a healthy metabolism through proper nutrition, physical activity, and lifestyle choices can optimize weight loss outcomes and overall well-being.

Discussion on why crash diets and extreme measures are not sustainable solutions.

Crash diets and extreme weight loss measures are often tempting for individuals seeking rapid results, but they are not sustainable solutions for long-term weight management. Here's a discussion on why crash diets and extreme measures are not sustainable:

- *Nutritional Deficiencies:* Crash diets typically involve severe calorie restriction and elimination of entire food groups, leading to nutrient deficiencies. Essential vitamins, minerals, and macronutrients are necessary for overall health and proper metabolic function. Depriving the body of these nutrients can lead to fatigue, weakness, compromised immune function, and other health issues.

- *Muscle Loss:* Rapid weight loss from crash diets often results in significant muscle loss along with fat loss. This is detrimental because muscle tissue plays a crucial role in metabolic rate. Losing muscle mass can slow down metabolism, making it harder to maintain weight loss in the long term.

- *Metabolic Adaptation:* Extreme calorie restriction can trigger metabolic adaptations aimed at conserving energy. The body may enter "starvation mode," slowing down metabolism to preserve energy stores and promote survival. As a result, weight loss may plateau, and further reductions in calorie intake become necessary to continue losing weight, leading to a cycle of deprivation and metabolic slowdown.

- *Loss of Lean Body Mass:* Crash diets primarily target fat stores for energy, but they can also lead to the loss of lean body mass, including muscle and organ tissue. This can compromise overall health and increase the risk of metabolic disorders, such as insulin resistance and fatty liver disease.

- *Negative Psychological Effects:* Crash diets often promote a restrictive and all-or-nothing approach to eating, which can lead to feelings of deprivation, guilt, and shame surrounding food. This can contribute to disordered eating patterns, emotional distress, and a dysfunctional relationship with food.

- *Weight Regain:* Research consistently shows that the majority of individuals who lose weight through crash diets or extreme measures regain the weight over time. This is due to physiological and psychological factors, including metabolic adaptations, hormonal changes, and unsustainable dietary practices. Without addressing the underlying behaviors and lifestyle factors contributing to weight gain, long-term weight maintenance is unlikely.

- ***Risk of Health Complications:*** Crash diets and extreme weight loss measures can pose serious health risks, including electrolyte imbalances, dehydration, gallstones, and cardiac complications. These risks may outweigh the short-term benefits of rapid weight loss.

While crash diets and extreme measures may yield quick results in the short term, they are not sustainable or healthy approaches to weight management. Sustainable weight loss requires a balanced, evidence-based approach that prioritizes whole foods, regular physical activity, behavioral changes, and gradual progress over time. It's essential to focus on long-term health and well-being rather than short-term fixes that can compromise overall health and lead to weight regain.

CHAPTER 2: EAT LESS, LOSE MORE

Strategies for reducing calorie intake without feeling deprived.

Reducing calorie intake without feeling deprived is key to sustainable weight loss and long-term success.

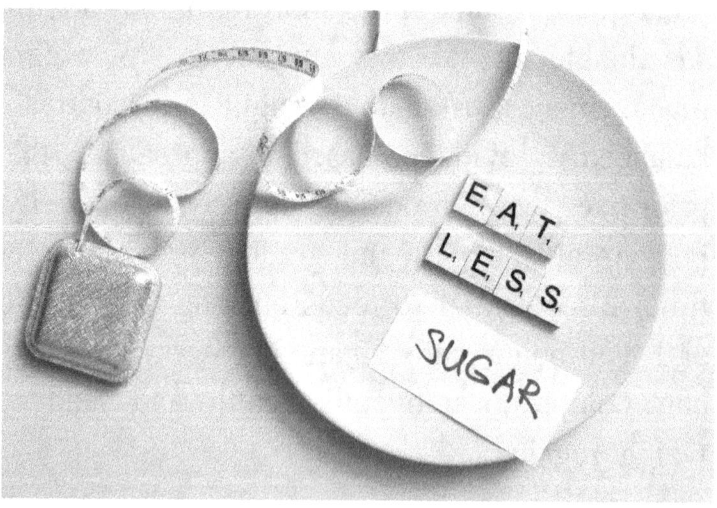

Here are some strategies to achieve this goal:

- *Focus on Whole Foods:* Fill your plate with nutrient-dense, whole foods such as fruits, vegetables, lean proteins, whole grains, and healthy fats. These foods are typically lower in calories and higher in fiber, which can help you feel full and satisfied.

- *Practice Portion Control:* Be mindful of portion sizes by using smaller plates, bowls, and utensils. Aim to fill half your plate with non-starchy vegetables, one-quarter with lean protein, and one-quarter with whole grains or starchy vegetables.

- *Eat Regularly:* Establish a consistent eating schedule with three balanced meals and healthy snacks throughout the day. This can help prevent excessive hunger and reduce the likelihood of overeating at mealtimes.

- ***Stay Hydrated:*** Drink plenty of water throughout the day, as thirst can sometimes be mistaken for hunger. Opt for water or other low-calorie beverages instead of sugary drinks or high-calorie beverages.

- ***Choose Low-Calorie Options:*** Swap high-calorie foods for lower-calorie alternatives whenever possible. For example, choose air-popped popcorn instead of chips, plain Greek yogurt instead of flavored yogurt, and fresh fruit instead of sugary snacks.

- ***Mindful Eating:*** Pay attention to your hunger and fullness cues by eating slowly, savoring each bite, and stopping when you feel satisfied. Avoid eating in front of the TV or computer, as this can lead to mindless overeating.

- ***Plan and Prep Meals:*** Take time to plan and prepare healthy meals and snacks in advance. This can help you make better food choices and avoid impulsive eating or relying on convenience foods.

- ***Include Protein and Fiber:*** Incorporate protein-rich foods such as lean meats, poultry, fish, tofu, beans, and legumes into your meals and snacks. Protein helps promote feelings of fullness and satisfaction. Additionally, include high-fiber foods like fruits, vegetables, whole grains, and legumes, which can also help you feel fuller for longer.

- ***Be Flexible:*** Allow yourself to enjoy your favorite foods in moderation. Restricting certain foods entirely can lead to feelings of deprivation and may ultimately backfire. Instead, practice moderation and portion control when indulging in treats or higher-calorie foods.

- ***Stay Active:*** Regular physical activity not only burns calories but can also help regulate appetite and improve mood. Find activities you enjoy and make them a regular part of your routine.

- ***Keep a Food Journal:*** Track your food intake and monitor your progress towards your calorie goals. This can help you identify patterns, make adjustments, and stay accountable.

By implementing these strategies, you can reduce calorie intake without feeling deprived and achieve sustainable weight loss while still enjoying delicious and satisfying meals. Remember to focus on progress, not perfection, and prioritize overall health and well-being.

Tips for portion control, mindful eating, and avoiding common pitfalls.

Portion control and mindful eating are crucial components of a healthy and balanced approach to nutrition. By practicing these habits, you can better manage your calorie intake, improve digestion, and cultivate a healthier relationship with food. Here are some tips for portion control, mindful eating, and avoiding common pitfalls:

Use Smaller Plates and Bowls: Opting for smaller dishware can naturally limit portion sizes without sacrificing satisfaction. The visual cue of a full plate can trick your brain into feeling content with less food. Reserve larger plates for salads and vegetables to encourage filling up on lower-calorie options.

Measure Portions: While it might seem tedious at first, measuring portions can provide valuable insight into appropriate serving sizes. Use measuring cups, spoons, or a food scale to accurately portion out foods, especially calorie-dense items like nuts, oils, and grains. Over time, you'll develop a better sense of portion sizes and may not need to measure as frequently.

Follow the Plate Method: Divide your plate into sections to ensure a balanced meal. Fill half of your plate with non-starchy vegetables like leafy greens, broccoli, or peppers. Allocate one-quarter of the plate to lean proteins such as chicken breast, fish, tofu, or beans. Reserve the remaining quarter for whole grains like brown rice, quinoa, or whole-wheat pasta. This method provides a variety of nutrients while controlling portion sizes.

Practice the Hand Method: Your hand can serve as a simple tool for estimating portion sizes, especially when you don't have measuring tools available. For example, a serving of protein should be about the size of your palm, a serving of carbohydrates should be about the size of your fist, and a serving of fats should be about the size of your thumb.

Listen to Your Body: Tune in to your body's hunger and fullness signals. Eat when you're genuinely hungry and stop when you're comfortably satisfied, rather than when your plate is empty or the clock dictates. Take breaks between bites, chew slowly, and pay attention to the flavors, textures, and sensations of each mouthful. This mindful approach can prevent overeating and enhance the enjoyment of your meals.

Eat Slowly: Slow down the pace of your meals to give your body time to register fullness. Research suggests that eating slowly can lead to reduced calorie intake and increased feelings of satisfaction. Put your fork down between bites, engage in conversation, and savor the experience of eating. Aim to chew each mouthful thoroughly, aiming for 20-30 chews per bite.

Minimize Distractions: Avoid eating in front of screens or while multitasking, as distractions can lead to mindless eating and overconsumption. Instead, create a calm and enjoyable environment for meals by sitting down at a table, setting the table with care, and focusing on the sensory experience of eating. Engage your senses by appreciating the aroma, appearance, taste, and texture of your food.

Be Mindful of Emotional Eating: Be aware of the emotional triggers that may influence your eating habits. Practice alternative coping strategies for dealing with stress, boredom, sadness, or other emotions, such as going for a walk, practicing deep breathing exercises, journaling, or reaching out to a supportive friend or family member. By addressing the underlying emotions, you can reduce the urge to turn to food for comfort.

Plan Ahead: Prepare healthy snacks and meals in advance to avoid impulsive food choices when hunger strikes. Stock your kitchen with portioned-out snacks like fresh fruit, cut-up vegetables, yogurt, or nuts. Having nutritious options readily available can prevent you from reaching for less healthy alternatives when cravings strike. Additionally, plan your meals for the week ahead, including grocery shopping and meal prep, to ensure you have balanced and satisfying options on hand.

Be Kind to Yourself: Remember that developing healthy eating habits is a journey, not a destination. It's okay to indulge occasionally, and it's normal to have setbacks along the way. Avoid harsh self-criticism or guilt over minor slip-ups. Instead, focus on progress, not perfection, and celebrate your successes, no matter how small. Treat yourself with compassion and kindness as you navigate the ups and downs of your wellness journey.

By incorporating these tips into your daily routine, you can develop healthier eating habits, improve portion control, and enjoy a more balanced and mindful approach to food.

CHAPTER 3: THE POWER OF EXERCISE

Exercise is a fundamental aspect of human physiology, with profound effects on physical health, mental well-being, and overall quality of life. From boosting cardiovascular health and strengthening muscles to reducing stress and enhancing mood, the power of exercise extends far beyond the confines of the gym.

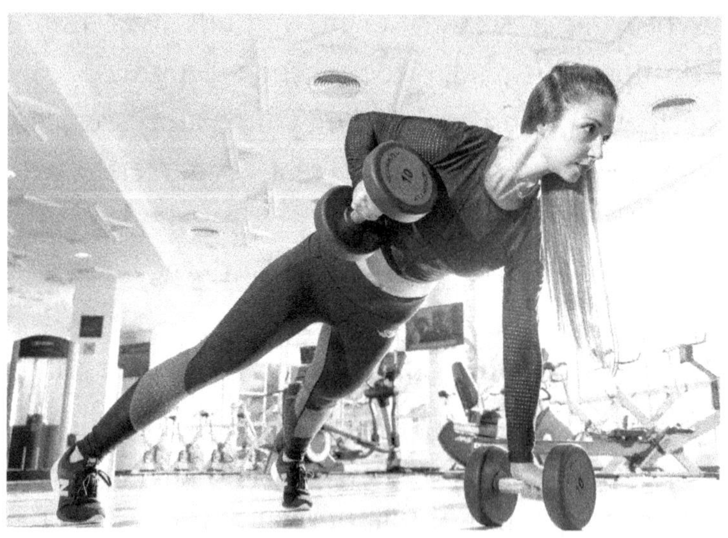

In this comprehensive exploration, we delve into the transformative impact of exercise on the mind, body, and soul, uncovering the myriad benefits that regular physical activity offers to individuals of all ages and backgrounds.

Physical Health Benefits:
- *Cardiovascular Health:* Regular exercise strengthens the heart muscle, improves blood circulation, and lowers blood pressure, reducing the risk of heart disease, stroke, and other cardiovascular conditions.

- *Weight Management:* Exercise helps regulate metabolism, burn calories, and build lean muscle mass, supporting weight loss and weight maintenance efforts.

- *Bone Health:* Weight-bearing exercises, such as walking, jogging, and resistance training, promote bone density and reduce the risk of osteoporosis and bone fractures.

- *Immune Function:* Moderate exercise enhances immune function by boosting circulation and promoting the production of immune cells, reducing the risk of infections and chronic diseases.

- *Chronic Disease Prevention:* Physical activity plays a crucial role in preventing and managing chronic conditions such as type 2 diabetes, hypertension, and certain types of cancer.

Mental Health Benefits:

- *Stress Reduction:* Exercise stimulates the release of endorphins, neurotransmitters that act as natural stress relievers, promoting relaxation and reducing feelings of anxiety and tension.

- *Mood Enhancement:* Regular physical activity increases levels of serotonin and dopamine, neurotransmitters associated with feelings of happiness and well-being, alleviating symptoms of depression and boosting mood.

- *Cognitive Function:* Exercise improves cognitive function, memory, and concentration by increasing blood flow to the brain and promoting the growth of new brain cells and connections.

- *Sleep Quality:* Physical activity regulates sleep patterns and promotes deeper, more restful sleep, leading to improved overall sleep quality and daytime alertness.

- *Self-Esteem:* Achieving fitness goals and experiencing improvements in physical appearance and performance can boost self-confidence and self-esteem, enhancing overall self-image and well-being.

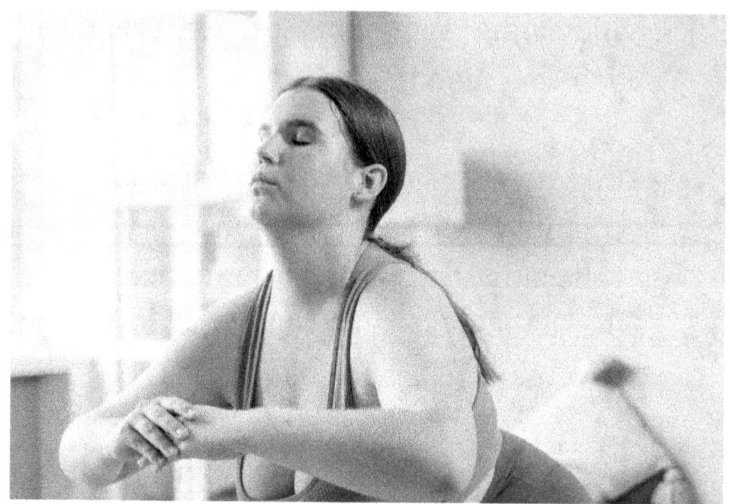

Social and Emotional Benefits:

- *Social Connection:* Exercise provides opportunities for social interaction and community engagement, fostering connections with others who share similar interests and goals.

- *Sense of Achievement:* Setting and achieving fitness goals, whether it's completing a race, mastering a new exercise, or reaching a personal best, instills a sense of accomplishment and pride.

- *Stress Relief:* Engaging in physical activities such as sports, dance, or yoga can serve as outlets for self-expression, creativity, and emotional release, helping individuals cope with life's challenges and pressures.

The power of exercise to transform lives cannot be overstated. From improving physical health and mental well-being to fostering social connections and enhancing quality of life, regular physical activity offers a multitude of benefits that extend far beyond the physical realm. By incorporating exercise into our daily routines and embracing an active lifestyle, we can unleash our full potential and embark on a journey towards a happier, healthier, and more fulfilling life.

Importance of physical activity in achieving and maintaining weight loss.

Physical activity is a cornerstone of successful weight loss efforts, playing a crucial role in both shedding excess pounds and maintaining a healthy body weight over the long term. In this discussion, we explore the importance of incorporating regular exercise into weight loss strategies, highlighting its numerous benefits for enhancing calorie expenditure, improving metabolic health, and supporting sustainable lifestyle changes.

Calorie Expenditure:

- Physical activity increases energy expenditure, helping individuals create a calorie deficit necessary for weight loss. Whether through aerobic exercises like running, cycling, or swimming, or strength training activities like weightlifting or bodyweight exercises, engaging in regular physical activity burns calories and contributes to overall energy balance.

- Higher intensity activities, such as interval training or HIIT (High-Intensity Interval Training), can elevate the body's metabolic rate even after exercise, resulting in greater calorie burn throughout the day.

Metabolic Health:
- Exercise improves metabolic health by enhancing insulin sensitivity and glucose metabolism, which are crucial for regulating blood sugar levels and preventing insulin resistance and type 2 diabetes.

- Resistance training, in particular, helps build lean muscle mass, which increases resting metabolic rate and promotes fat loss, even at rest. Muscle tissue requires more energy to maintain than fat tissue, leading to a higher overall metabolic rate.

- Regular physical activity also supports healthy lipid profiles, reducing levels of LDL (bad) cholesterol and triglycerides while increasing HDL (good) cholesterol, thereby lowering the risk of cardiovascular disease.

Appetite Regulation:

- Physical activity influences appetite regulation and satiety hormones, such as ghrelin and leptin, which help control hunger and food intake. Moderate exercise can suppress appetite in the short term, making it easier to adhere to a calorie-restricted diet.

- Additionally, engaging in regular exercise may improve food choices and reduce cravings for high-calorie, unhealthy foods, further supporting weight loss efforts.

Psychological and Behavioral Benefits:

- Exercise has numerous psychological and behavioral benefits that support weight loss success. It reduces stress, anxiety, and depression, which can trigger emotional eating and sabotage weight loss efforts.

- Regular physical activity improves mood, boosts self-esteem, and increases feelings of self-efficacy and motivation, all of which are essential for maintaining long-term adherence to healthy lifestyle changes.

- Participating in group exercise classes or team sports fosters social support and accountability, providing encouragement and camaraderie to individuals on their weight loss journey.

Physical activity is a critical component of achieving and maintaining weight loss. By incorporating regular exercise into daily routines, individuals can increase calorie expenditure, improve metabolic health, regulate appetite, and enhance psychological well-being, all of which contribute to successful long-term weight management. Whether through aerobic activities, strength training, or a combination of both, prioritizing physical activity is essential for reaching weight loss goals and sustaining a healthy lifestyle for years to come.

Different types of exercises and their benefits, including cardio, strength training, and flexibility exercises.

Exercise encompasses a wide range of activities, each offering unique benefits for physical health, mental well-being, and overall fitness. From cardiovascular workouts that improve endurance and heart health to strength training exercises that build muscle and bone density, and flexibility exercises that enhance mobility and reduce the risk of injury, incorporating a variety of exercise modalities into your fitness routine is essential for achieving comprehensive health and fitness goals. In this discussion, we explore the different types of exercises and their respective benefits.

Cardiovascular Exercise:

Cardiovascular exercise, also known as aerobic exercise, includes activities that elevate the heart rate and increase oxygen consumption over an extended period. Examples include walking, running, cycling, swimming, and dancing.

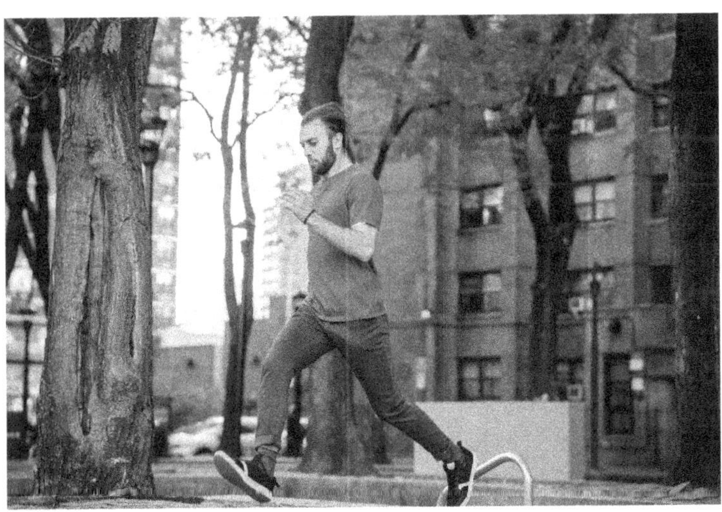

Benefits:

- Improves cardiovascular health by strengthening the heart muscle and improving blood circulation.

- Increases lung capacity and oxygen delivery to tissues, enhancing endurance and stamina.

- Helps burn calories and promote weight loss by increasing energy expenditure during and after exercise.

- Reduces the risk of chronic diseases such as heart disease, stroke, type 2 diabetes, and certain cancers.

- Boosts mood and reduces stress, anxiety, and symptoms of depression through the release of endorphins and other neurotransmitters.

Strength Training:

Strength training, also known as resistance training or weight training, involves using external resistance, such as free weights, resistance bands, or machines, to strengthen muscles and improve overall muscular fitness.

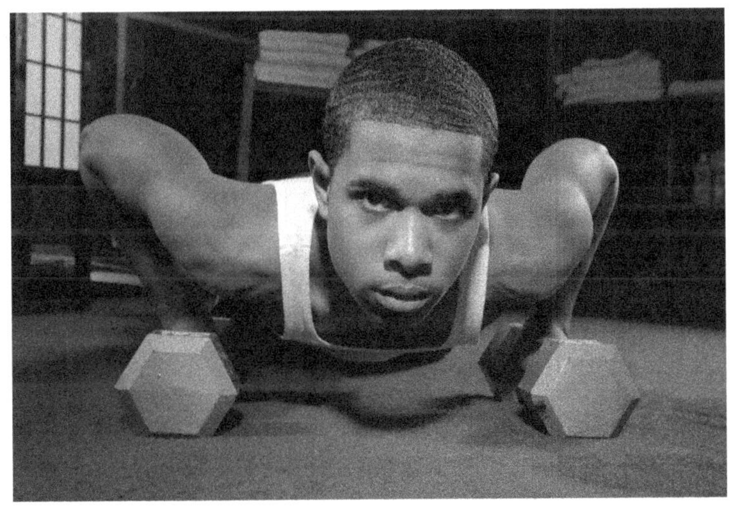

Benefits:

- Increases muscle mass and strength, leading to improvements in functional capacity, mobility, and balance.

- Boosts metabolism and promotes fat loss by increasing resting metabolic rate and promoting calorie expenditure, even at rest.

- Enhances bone density and reduces the risk of osteoporosis and bone fractures, particularly in older adults.

- Improves joint health and stability, reducing the risk of injury and enhancing athletic performance.

- Contributes to a toned and sculpted physique, improving body composition and enhancing self-confidence.

Flexibility and Mobility Exercises:

Flexibility and mobility exercises focus on improving joint range of motion, muscle flexibility, and overall mobility. Examples include stretching, yoga, Pilates, and mobility drills.

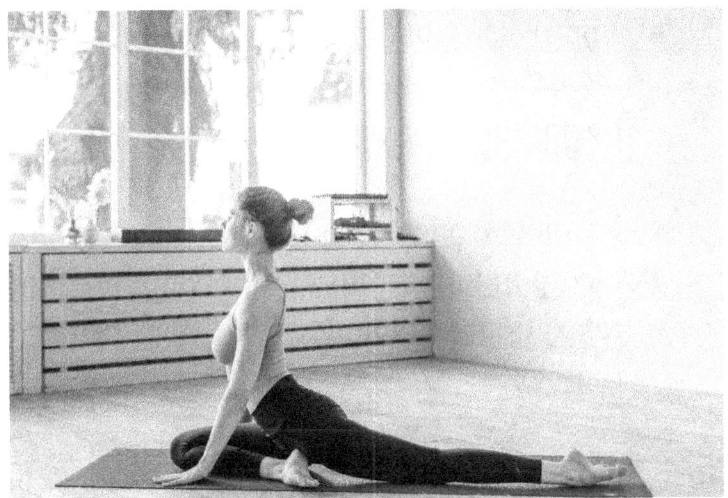

Benefits:

- Increases flexibility and joint range of motion, allowing for greater freedom of movement and improved functional capacity.

- Reduces the risk of injury by improving muscle elasticity and reducing muscle stiffness and tension.

- Enhances posture and alignment, reducing the risk of musculoskeletal imbalances and chronic pain.

- Improves athletic performance by increasing agility, coordination, and overall movement efficiency.

- Promotes relaxation and stress relief by incorporating mindful breathing and relaxation techniques into the exercise routine.

Incorporating a variety of exercises into your fitness regimen is essential for achieving comprehensive health and fitness goals. Cardiovascular exercise improves heart health and endurance, strength training builds muscle mass and bone density, and flexibility exercises enhance mobility and reduce the risk of injury. By incorporating these different types of exercises into your routine, you can optimize physical health, mental well-being, and overall fitness for a healthier, happier life.

CHAPTER 4: CREATING A SUSTAINABLE WORKOUT ROUTINE

Embarking on a fitness journey requires more than just sporadic bursts of activity; it necessitates the development of a sustainable workout routine that can be maintained over the long term. By establishing a balanced and adaptable plan that aligns with your goals, preferences, and lifestyle, you can cultivate habits that promote consistent progress and lasting results.

Creating a sustainable workout routine requires careful planning, patience, and dedication, but the rewards are well worth the effort. By setting realistic goals, choosing enjoyable activities, prioritizing variety and balance, and listening to your body, you can cultivate habits that support long-term fitness success and overall well-being. Remember to stay consistent, stay adaptable, and most importantly, enjoy the journey towards a healthier, happier you.

How to design a personalized exercise plan that fits your lifestyle and goals.

Designing a personalized exercise plan that fits your lifestyle and goals involves several key steps to ensure it is tailored to your individual needs, preferences, and circumstances. Here's a comprehensive guide to help you create a customized workout routine:

Assess Your Current Fitness Level:
- Begin by evaluating your current fitness level, including strength, cardiovascular endurance, flexibility, and mobility. This can be done through self-assessment exercises, fitness tests, or consultations with a fitness professional.

- Consider any existing health conditions, injuries, or physical limitations that may impact your exercise routine.

Set Specific and Realistic Goals:

- Determine your fitness goals, whether they are related to weight loss, muscle gain, improving endurance, enhancing flexibility, or overall health and well-being.

- Make your goals specific, measurable, attainable, relevant, and time-bound (SMART) to provide clarity and motivation for your exercise plan.

Identify Your Preferences and Lifestyle Factors:

- Consider your personal preferences, interests, and lifestyle when designing your workout routine. Choose activities and exercises that you enjoy and can realistically incorporate into your daily or weekly schedule.

- Take into account factors such as time constraints, availability of facilities or equipment, budget considerations, and social support systems.

Select Appropriate Types of Exercise:
- Choose a variety of exercises that align with your goals and preferences, including cardiovascular activities, strength training exercises, flexibility and mobility drills, and recreational activities.

- Mix and match different types of exercise to keep your routine engaging and challenging, while also targeting different muscle groups and energy systems.

Determine Frequency, Duration, and Intensity:
- Decide how often you will exercise each week and for how long. Aim for at least 150 minutes of moderate-intensity aerobic

activity or 75 minutes of vigorous-intensity aerobic activity per week, along with muscle-strengthening activities on two or more days.

- Gradually increase the intensity, duration, and frequency of your workouts as your fitness level improves, while also allowing for adequate rest and recovery between sessions.

Create a Structured Workout Plan:
- Develop a structured workout plan that outlines the specific exercises, sets, repetitions, and rest periods for each workout session.

- Incorporate a warm-up and cool-down period into each workout to prepare your body for exercise and prevent injury.

Consider Cross-Training and Periodization:
- Incorporate cross-training into your exercise plan by including a variety of

activities and movements to prevent boredom, overuse injuries, and plateaus.

- Implement periodization techniques, such as varying the intensity, volume, and frequency of your workouts over time, to optimize progress and prevent burnout.

Monitor Progress and Adjust as Needed:

- Keep track of your progress by recording your workouts, tracking changes in fitness metrics, and regularly reassessing your goals.

- Be flexible and willing to adjust your exercise plan based on changes in your schedule, preferences, or fitness level. Experiment with different exercises, routines, and training methods to find what works best for you.

Seek Professional Guidance if Needed:

- Consider seeking guidance from a certified personal trainer, fitness coach, or exercise physiologist to help you design a personalized exercise plan that aligns with your goals and abilities.

- A fitness professional can provide expert advice, motivation, accountability, and support to help you reach your fitness goals safely and effectively.

Stay Consistent and Enjoy the Process:
- Consistency is key to success, so make exercise a regular part of your routine and prioritize it just like any other important commitment in your life.
- Focus on enjoying the process of exercise and celebrating small victories along the way. Remember that progress takes time, patience, and dedication, so stay committed to your goals and keep moving forward.

By following these steps and tailoring your exercise plan to fit your lifestyle and goals, you can create a personalized workout routine that is both effective and sustainable in the long term. Remember to listen to your body, stay flexible, and make adjustments as needed to ensure continued progress and enjoyment of your fitness journey.

Overcoming barriers to exercise and staying motivated for the long term.

Overcoming barriers to exercise and staying motivated for the long term is essential for achieving and maintaining a healthy lifestyle.

Identifying Common Barriers to Exercise:
- *Lack of Time:* Busy schedules and competing priorities can make it challenging to find time for exercise.

- *Lack of Motivation:* Feelings of boredom, fatigue, or discouragement can sap motivation and enthusiasm for exercise.

- *Physical Limitations:* Health issues, injuries, or physical discomfort may hinder participation in certain types of exercise.

- *Environmental Factors:* Limited access to exercise facilities, inclement weather, or unsafe neighborhoods can pose obstacles to physical activity.

- *Lack of Social Support:* A lack of encouragement or accountability from friends, family, or peers can make it difficult to stay motivated.

Here are some strategies to help you overcome common obstacles and sustain your motivation:

Strategies for Overcoming Barriers:

- *Prioritize Exercise:* Make exercise a non-negotiable part of your daily or weekly routine by scheduling it in advance and treating it as an important commitment.

- *Set Realistic Goals:* Break down your fitness goals into smaller, achievable milestones, and celebrate your progress along the way.

- *Find Activities You Enjoy:* Choose exercises and activities that you genuinely enjoy and look forward to, whether it's dancing, hiking, swimming, or playing sports.

- *Make Exercise Convenient:* Find ways to integrate physical activity into your daily life, such as taking the stairs instead of the elevator, walking or biking to work, or exercising at home with online workout videos.

- *Be Flexible:* Be willing to adapt your exercise routine to accommodate changes in your schedule, preferences, or circumstances. Explore different types of exercise and find what works best for you.

- *Seek Social Support:* Surround yourself with supportive friends, family members, or workout buddies who can encourage and motivate you on your fitness journey. Joining group exercise classes or online fitness communities can also provide accountability and camaraderie.

- *Focus on the Benefits:* Remind yourself of the numerous benefits of exercise, including improved health, increased energy, stress relief, better mood, and enhanced self-confidence.

- *Practice Self-Compassion:* Be kind to yourself and acknowledge that setbacks are a normal part of the journey. Instead of dwelling on mistakes or missed workouts, focus on getting back on track and moving forward.

- *Reward Yourself:* Treat yourself to small rewards or incentives for reaching milestones or sticking to your exercise routine. This could be anything from a relaxing massage to a new workout outfit or a healthy meal at your favorite restaurant.

Cultivating Long-Term Motivation:

- *Find Your Why:* Identify your deeper reasons for wanting to achieve weight loss and improve your health. Whether it's to feel more confident, set a positive example for your family, or live a longer, healthier life, connecting with your underlying motivations can help sustain your commitment to exercise.

- *Visualize Success:* Create a mental image of yourself achieving your fitness goals and visualize the positive changes and benefits that come with it. This can help reinforce your commitment and keep you motivated during challenging times.

- *Track Your Progress:* Keep track of your workouts, measurements, and achievements to monitor your progress over time. Seeing tangible results can provide motivation and reinforce the importance of your efforts.

- *Mix It Up:* Keep your workouts interesting and engaging by varying your routine, trying new activities, and setting new challenges for yourself. This prevents boredom and keeps you mentally stimulated and motivated to continue exercising.

- *Celebrate Milestones:* Celebrate your successes and milestones along the way, whether it's reaching a new personal best, completing a challenging workout, or sticking to your exercise routine for a certain period. Acknowledging your achievements boosts confidence and reinforces positive habits.

Overcoming barriers to exercise and sustaining motivation for long-term weight loss success requires commitment, perseverance, and a willingness to adapt. By identifying common obstacles, implementing strategies to overcome them, and cultivating long-term motivation, you can stay on track with your fitness goals and achieve lasting results. Remember that progress takes time, patience, and consistency, so stay focused, stay positive, and keep moving forward on your journey to better health and well-being.

CHAPTER 5: FINDING BALANCE IN YOUR DIET

Finding balance in your diet is essential for maintaining overall health and well-being. Here are some tips to help you achieve a balanced and nutritious diet:

Include a Variety of Foods:
Aim to incorporate a wide range of foods from all food groups into your diet, including fruits, vegetables, whole grains, lean proteins, and healthy fats. Variety ensures that you get a diverse array of nutrients and phytochemicals that support optimal health.

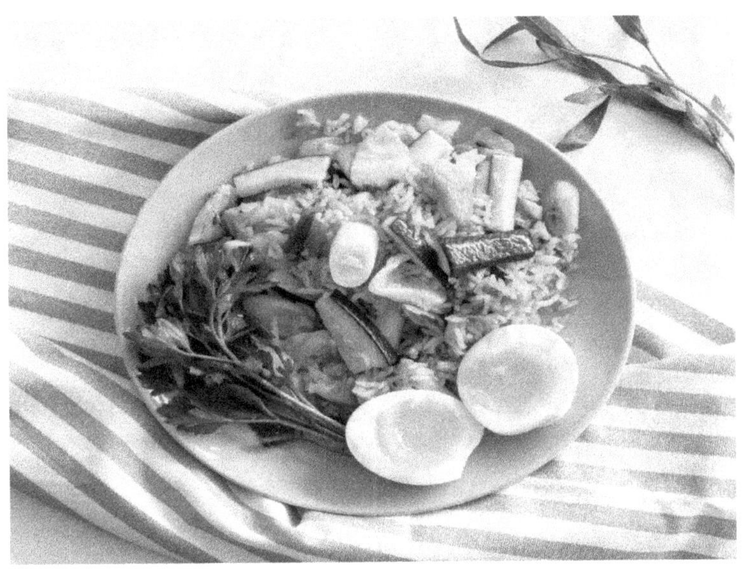

Focus on Whole Foods:

Choose whole, minimally processed foods whenever possible. Whole foods are rich in nutrients, fiber, and antioxidants, and they provide sustained energy while supporting overall health. Examples include fruits, vegetables, whole grains, legumes, nuts, seeds, lean proteins, and dairy products.

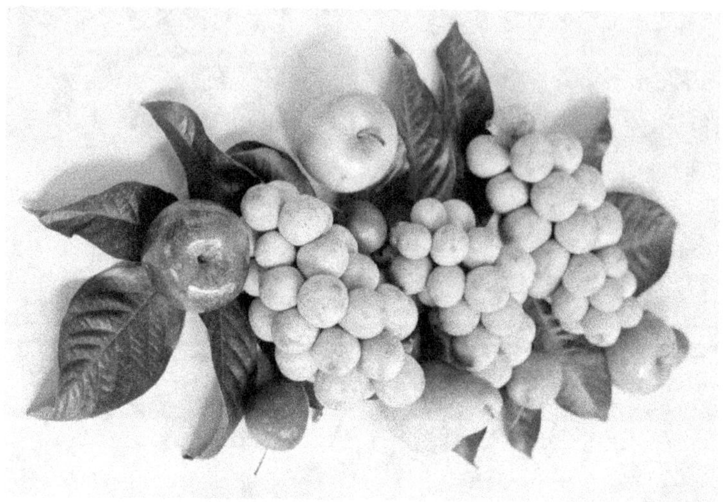

Practice Portion Control:

Be mindful of portion sizes and avoid overeating. Use visual cues, such as the size of your palm or a deck of cards, to estimate appropriate portion sizes for different food groups. Eating smaller, more frequent meals throughout the day can help prevent excessive calorie intake and promote better digestion.

Balance Macronutrients:
Ensure that your meals include a balance of carbohydrates, proteins, and fats. Carbohydrates provide energy, proteins support muscle growth and repair, and fats are essential for hormone production and nutrient absorption. Aim to include a source of each macronutrient in every meal for optimal balance and satiety.

Prioritize Plant-Based Foods:
Incorporate plenty of plant-based foods into your diet, including fruits, vegetables, legumes, nuts, seeds, and whole grains. Plant-based foods are rich in fiber, vitamins, minerals, and antioxidants, and they can help lower the risk of chronic diseases such as heart disease, diabetes, and certain cancers.

Limit Added Sugars and Processed Foods:
Minimize your intake of added sugars, refined grains, and processed foods, which can contribute to weight gain, inflammation, and chronic disease. Choose whole, nutrient-dense

foods over sugary snacks, desserts, and highly processed convenience foods.

Stay Hydrated:
Drink plenty of water throughout the day to stay hydrated and support optimal bodily functions. Aim for at least eight glasses of water per day, and consider hydrating with herbal teas, infused water, or fresh fruits and vegetables.

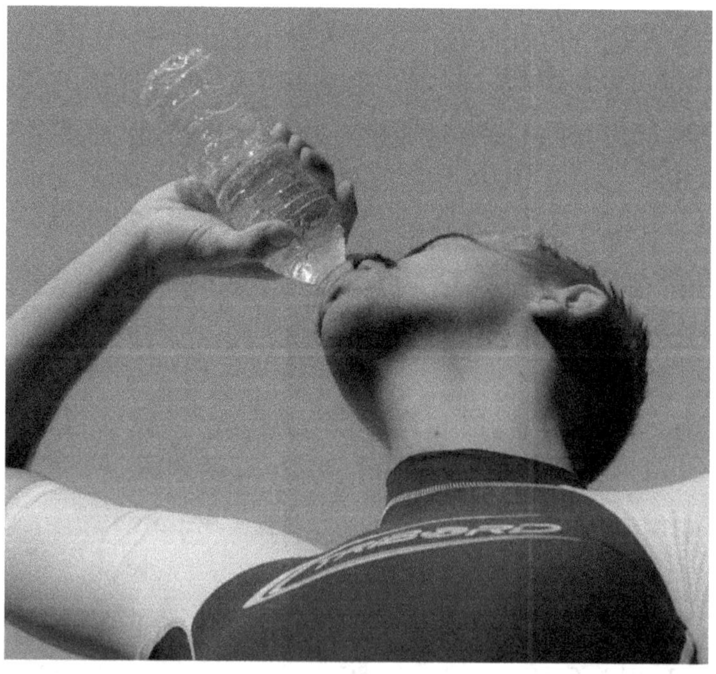

Practice Mindful Eating:
Pay attention to your hunger and fullness cues, and eat slowly and mindfully to fully enjoy and appreciate your meals. Avoid distractions such as television or smartphones while eating, and savor the flavors, textures, and aromas of your food.

Plan and Prepare Meals Ahead of Time:
Plan your meals and snacks in advance to ensure that you have balanced, nutritious options readily available. Meal prepping can help save time and money, reduce food waste, and prevent impulsive food choices when hunger strikes.

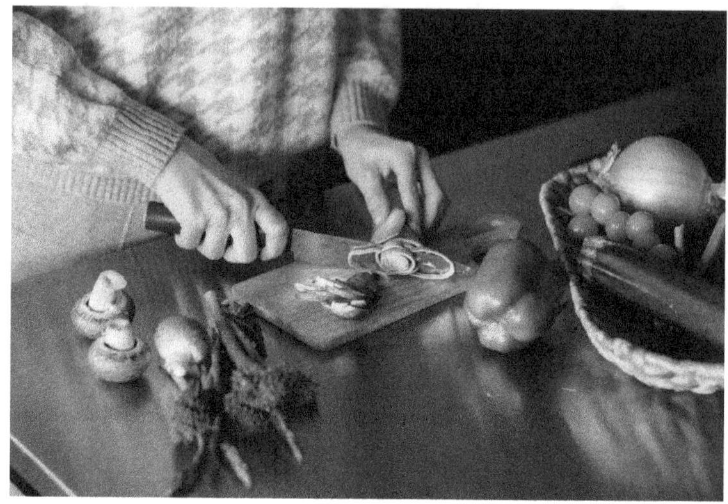

Be Flexible and Enjoy Treats in Moderation:
Allow yourself to enjoy indulgent foods and treats occasionally, but do so in moderation. Depriving yourself of your favorite foods can lead to feelings of deprivation and ultimately sabotage your efforts to maintain a balanced diet. Instead, aim for balance and moderation in your food choices, and focus on nourishing your body with nutrient-dense foods most of the time. Finding balance in your diet is a lifelong journey that requires mindful choices, experimentation, and self-awareness. By following these tips and listening to your body's needs, you can cultivate

a healthy relationship with food and achieve optimal health and well-being.

The role of macronutrients (carbohydrates, proteins, fats) in a balanced diet.

Macronutrients—carbohydrates, proteins, and fats—are the primary components of our diet, providing the energy and essential nutrients needed for optimal health and well-being. Each macronutrient plays a distinct role in the body and is essential for supporting various physiological functions. In this discussion, we explore the importance of macronutrients in achieving a balanced diet and their roles in promoting overall health.

Carbohydrates:
Carbohydrates are the body's primary source of energy, providing fuel for brain function, physical activity, and metabolic processes.

Main sources of carbohydrates include grains, fruits, vegetables, legumes, and dairy products.

Carbohydrates are classified into simple and complex carbohydrates based on their chemical structure and how quickly they are digested and absorbed.

Simple carbohydrates, such as sugars found in fruits, honey, and processed foods, provide quick energy but can cause rapid spikes and crashes in blood sugar levels.

Complex carbohydrates, found in whole grains, legumes, and starchy vegetables, provide sustained energy and are rich in fiber, vitamins, and minerals.

Including a variety of carbohydrates in your diet, with an emphasis on whole, unprocessed sources, supports energy balance, blood sugar regulation, and digestive health.

Proteins:

Proteins are essential for building and repairing tissues, synthesizing enzymes and hormones, and supporting immune function.

Main sources of protein include meat, poultry, fish, eggs, dairy products, legumes, nuts, seeds, and soy products.

Proteins are made up of amino acids, which are often referred to as the building blocks of life. There are 20 different amino acids, nine of which are considered essential because the body cannot produce them and must be obtained from the diet.

Consuming an adequate amount of high-quality protein supports muscle growth, recovery, and maintenance, as well as satiety and weight management.

Aim to include a variety of protein sources in your diet to ensure you get all essential amino acids and optimize overall protein intake.

Fats:

Fats are essential for providing energy, insulating organs, supporting cell growth, and absorbing fat-soluble vitamins (A, D, E, K).

Main sources of fats include oils, butter, avocados, nuts, seeds, fatty fish, and dairy products.

Fats are classified into saturated, unsaturated (monounsaturated and polyunsaturated), and trans fats based on their chemical structure and health effects.

Unsaturated fats, found in plant-based oils, nuts, seeds, and fatty fish, are considered heart-healthy and can help reduce the risk of cardiovascular disease.

Saturated fats, found in animal products and some plant oils, should be consumed in moderation to maintain heart health.

Trans fats, found in partially hydrogenated oils used in processed foods, should be avoided as they increase the risk of heart disease.

Including a balance of healthy fats in your diet supports brain function, hormone production, and overall cellular health.

Macronutrients—carbohydrates, proteins, and fats—play crucial roles in supporting energy metabolism, tissue repair, immune function, and overall health. Achieving a balanced diet that includes a variety of whole, nutrient-dense foods from each macronutrient group is essential for meeting nutritional needs, promoting satiety, and maintaining optimal health and well-being. By understanding the roles of macronutrients and making informed dietary choices, you can support your body's needs and enjoy a balanced and nutritious diet for long-term health.

Tips for incorporating a variety of foods to ensure nutritional adequacy.

Incorporating a variety of foods into your diet is key to ensuring nutritional adequacy and promoting overall health and well-being. Here are some tips to help you achieve dietary diversity and maximize nutrient intake:

Include a Rainbow of Fruits and Vegetables:

- Aim to consume a wide variety of fruits and vegetables of different colors, as each color indicates a unique set of vitamins, minerals, antioxidants, and phytochemicals.

- Include a mix of leafy greens, cruciferous vegetables, root vegetables, berries, citrus fruits, and other seasonal produce to provide a diverse array of nutrients and health-promoting compounds.

Incorporate Whole Grains:

- Choose whole grains such as brown rice, quinoa, barley, oats, whole wheat, and bulgur over refined grains like white rice and white bread.

- Experiment with different types of whole grains to add texture and flavor to your meals, such as using quinoa in salads, bulgur in pilafs, or oats in breakfast porridge.

Include a Variety of Protein Sources:

- Incorporate a mix of animal-based and plant-based protein sources into your diet, such as lean meats, poultry, fish, eggs, dairy products, legumes, tofu, tempeh, seitan, nuts, and seeds.

- Rotate your protein sources throughout the week to ensure you get a diverse array of amino acids and micronutrients.

Choose Healthy Fats:

- Include a variety of healthy fats in your diet from sources such as avocados, nuts, seeds, olive oil, coconut oil, fatty fish (salmon, mackerel, sardines), and flaxseeds.

- Use different types of oils for cooking, salad dressings, and dips to add flavor and diversity to your meals.

Experiment with Herbs and Spices:

- Use herbs, spices, and aromatic ingredients to enhance the flavor of your dishes without adding excess salt, sugar, or unhealthy fats.

- Experiment with different flavor combinations and ethnic cuisines to keep your meals interesting and flavorful.

Include Dairy or Dairy Alternatives:

- If you consume dairy, choose a variety of dairy products such as milk, yogurt, cheese, and kefir to ensure you get a mix of nutrients like calcium, vitamin D, and protein.

- If you're lactose intolerant or follow a vegan diet, opt for fortified plant-based alternatives like almond milk, soy yogurt, or cashew cheese.

Snack Smartly:

- Choose nutrient-dense snacks that provide a mix of macronutrients and micronutrients, such as fresh fruit with nut butter, Greek yogurt with berries, raw vegetables with hummus, or whole-grain crackers with cheese.

- Keep a variety of healthy snacks on hand to satisfy cravings and prevent mindless munching on less nutritious options.

Plan Balanced Meals:

- When planning meals, aim to include a variety of foods from different food groups, including fruits, vegetables, whole grains, lean proteins, and healthy fats.

- Use the MyPlate or Healthy Eating Plate guidelines as a visual tool to ensure your meals are balanced and nutritionally adequate.

By incorporating a diverse array of foods into your diet, you can ensure that you're meeting your nutritional needs and enjoying a wide range of flavors, textures, and nutrients that support optimal health and well-being. Experiment with new foods, flavors, and cuisines to keep your meals exciting and satisfying while reaping the benefits of a varied and nutrient-rich diet.

CHAPTER 6: BUILDING HEALTHY EATING HABITS

Strategies for meal planning, grocery shopping, and preparing nutritious meals.

Creating a well-rounded approach to meal planning, grocery shopping, and meal preparation is essential for maintaining a balanced and nutritious diet.

Here are strategies to help you effectively manage these aspects of healthy eating:

Meal Planning:
- Set aside dedicated time each week to plan your meals for the upcoming days. Consider factors such as your schedule, dietary preferences, and nutritional needs.

- Start by creating a list of meals for breakfast, lunch, dinner, and snacks. Aim for variety and balance, incorporating different food groups and flavors.

- Utilize online resources, cookbooks, or meal planning apps for inspiration and recipe ideas. Consider batch cooking or preparing meals in advance to save time during busy weekdays.

- Keep your meal plan flexible to accommodate changes or unexpected events. Allow for some flexibility and spontaneity while maintaining a general structure.

Grocery Shopping:
- Before heading to the grocery store, review your meal plan and create a shopping list based on the ingredients you need. Organize your list by food

categories to streamline your shopping trip.

- Stick to the perimeter of the grocery store where fresh produce, lean proteins, dairy, and whole grains are typically located. Limit purchases of processed and packaged foods from the inner aisles.

- Choose seasonal fruits and vegetables, which tend to be fresher, more flavorful, and more affordable. Opt for organic options when possible, especially for produce with higher pesticide residue levels.

- Read food labels carefully and compare nutritional information to make informed choices. Look for products with minimal added sugars, sodium, and unhealthy fats, and prioritize whole, unprocessed foods.

- Consider shopping online or using grocery delivery services for added convenience and efficiency, especially if time or mobility is limited.

Meal Preparation:

- Dedicate time each week to meal preparation to ensure that healthy options are readily available when hunger strikes. Set aside a few hours to chop vegetables, cook grains, and prepare protein sources in bulk.

- Use versatile ingredients that can be repurposed into multiple meals throughout the week. For example, roast a batch of vegetables to use in salads, grain bowls, or stir-fries.

- Invest in time-saving kitchen tools and appliances such as a slow cooker, Instant Pot, or food processor to simplify meal preparation and cooking.

- Store prepared ingredients in portioned containers or reusable bags for easy grab-and-go options. Label containers with the date and contents to track freshness and prevent food waste.

- Get creative with meal prep by experimenting with different flavors, cuisines, and cooking techniques. Incorporate herbs, spices, and marinades to add variety and depth to your meals.

By implementing these strategies for meal planning, grocery shopping, and meal preparation, you can streamline the process of making nutritious meals and set yourself up for success in maintaining a healthy diet. Remember to stay flexible, listen to your body's hunger and fullness cues, and enjoy the process of nourishing yourself with delicious and wholesome foods.

How to navigate social situations and dining out while sticking to your weight loss goals.

Navigating social situations and dining out while adhering to weight loss goals can present challenges, but with mindful planning and strategic choices, it's entirely achievable. Here are some tips to help you stay on track while enjoying social gatherings and restaurant meals:

Plan Ahead:

Review the restaurant menu online in advance to identify healthier options and plan your meal choices accordingly. Look for dishes that are grilled, steamed, baked, or broiled rather than fried or heavily sautéed.

If possible, suggest restaurants that offer a variety of nutritious options, such as salad bars, build-your-own-bowl establishments, or venues with customizable menu items.

Eat a light, balanced snack before heading out to curb hunger and prevent overeating when faced with tempting food choices.

Practice Portion Control:

Be mindful of portion sizes and avoid the temptation to indulge in oversized portions or all-you-can-eat buffets. Consider sharing an entrée with a friend or requesting a half portion to control portion sizes.

Ask for a to-go container when your meal is served and portion out a suitable amount of food to enjoy, saving the rest for another meal.

Make Smart Substitutions:

Opt for healthier cooking methods such as grilling, steaming, or baking instead of frying. Ask for sauces, dressings, and condiments on the side to control the amount you consume.

Substitute high-calorie or high-fat ingredients with healthier alternatives whenever possible. For example, choose whole-grain options instead of refined grains and swap out creamy sauces for tomato-based or vinaigrette dressings.

Load Up on Vegetables:

Prioritize vegetable-based dishes or side dishes to fill up on fiber-rich, low-calorie foods that provide volume and satiety without excess calories.

Start your meal with a salad or vegetable-based soup to help curb hunger and prevent overeating during the main course.

Mindful Eating:

Eat slowly and savor each bite, paying attention to hunger and fullness cues. Put down your fork between bites, engage in conversation, and enjoy the social aspect of dining out without rushing through your meal.

Pause halfway through your meal to assess your hunger and satisfaction levels. Consider whether you're truly enjoying the food or simply eating out of habit or social pressure.

Limit Alcohol Consumption:

Be mindful of liquid calories from alcoholic beverages, sugary cocktails, and high-calorie mixed drinks. Opt for lighter options such as wine spritzers, light beer, or spirits mixed with club soda and fresh lime.

Alternate alcoholic drinks with water or other non-caloric beverages to stay hydrated and prevent excessive calorie intake.

Stay Flexible and Forgiving:

Remember that occasional indulgences are a normal part of life, and it's okay to enjoy your favorite foods in moderation. Avoid feelings of guilt or deprivation by practicing self-compassion and staying flexible with your eating habits.

If you do overindulge at a social gathering or restaurant meal, forgive yourself and move on. Focus on making healthier choices at your next meal and getting back on track with your weight loss goals.

By incorporating these strategies into your approach to social situations and dining out, you can enjoy the company of friends and family while staying true to your commitment to weight loss and overall health. Remember that balance, moderation, and mindfulness are key to long-term success, and celebrate your progress and accomplishments along the way.

CHAPTER 7: MIND-BODY CONNECTION

Exploring the link between emotions, stress, and eating habits.

In the intricate web of human experience, the connection between emotions, stress, and eating habits plays a significant role in shaping our relationship with food and overall well-being. Understanding how our emotional state and stress levels influence our eating behaviors is crucial for promoting healthy habits and preventing issues such as emotional eating, binge eating, and disordered eating patterns. In this exploration, we delve into the complex interplay between emotions, stress, and eating habits, shedding light on the psychological and physiological mechanisms at play and offering insights into how we can foster a more balanced and mindful approach to nourishing our bodies.

Emotional Eating:

Emotional eating refers to the tendency to turn to food for comfort, distraction, or relief from negative emotions such as stress, anxiety, boredom, or sadness.

Emotional triggers can lead to cravings for specific foods, often high in sugar, fat, or salt, which are perceived as soothing or rewarding.

Emotional eating can create a cycle of guilt, shame, and further emotional distress, perpetuating unhealthy eating habits and undermining efforts to maintain a balanced diet.

Stress Eating:

Stress eating, also known as "stress-induced eating" or "stress snacking," involves consuming food in response to heightened stress levels or emotional tension.

Stress triggers the release of cortisol, a hormone that stimulates appetite and cravings for high-calorie, comfort foods.

Chronic stress can disrupt appetite regulation and lead to overeating, particularly of foods that provide temporary relief from stress but offer little nutritional value.

Coping Mechanisms:
Food often serves as a coping mechanism for managing difficult emotions or stressful situations, providing temporary comfort or distraction from underlying issues.

Other coping strategies, such as mindfulness, relaxation techniques, physical activity, or seeking social support, can offer healthier alternatives to managing stress and emotional distress.

Mindful Eating:

Mindful eating involves paying attention to the sensory experience of eating, including taste, texture, and smell, without judgment or distraction.

By cultivating mindfulness around eating, individuals can become more attuned to their hunger and fullness cues, making it easier to differentiate between physical hunger and emotional hunger.

Practicing mindful eating can help break the cycle of emotional and stress eating, promoting greater awareness, satisfaction, and enjoyment of food.

Strategies for Healthy Eating:

Developing healthy coping mechanisms for managing emotions and stress, such as engaging in regular physical activity, practicing relaxation techniques, journaling, or seeking professional support.

Building a supportive environment that fosters healthy eating habits, including stocking nutritious foods, meal planning, and creating structured mealtimes.

Cultivating self-awareness and emotional resilience to better understand and manage triggers for emotional and stress eating, and developing positive coping strategies to address underlying needs.

The link between emotions, stress, and eating habits is a multifaceted phenomenon that requires a holistic approach to address effectively. By recognizing the influence of emotions and stress on our eating behaviors and implementing strategies for mindful eating and stress management, we can foster a healthier relationship with food and nourish our bodies in ways that promote overall well-being and vitality.

Techniques for managing stress and emotional eating to support weight loss efforts.

Stress and emotional eating can derail weight loss efforts by triggering cravings for unhealthy foods and leading to overeating. By learning to manage stress and emotional eating effectively, individuals can support their weight loss journey and cultivate healthier habits. Here are techniques to help manage stress and emotional eating, empowering individuals to make mindful choices and achieve their weight loss goals.

Stress Management Techniques:

- Practice relaxation techniques such as deep breathing exercises, progressive muscle relaxation, or guided imagery to reduce stress levels and promote relaxation.

- Engage in regular physical activity, such as walking, jogging, yoga, or dancing, to release tension, boost mood, and alleviate stress.

- Incorporate mindfulness practices, such as meditation or mindfulness meditation, to cultivate present-moment awareness and reduce stress reactivity.

- Prioritize self-care activities that promote relaxation and well-being, such as taking a warm bath, listening to calming music, or spending time in nature.

Emotional Regulation Strategies:
- Identify triggers for emotional eating, such as boredom, loneliness, sadness, or anxiety, and develop alternative coping mechanisms to address underlying emotions.

- Practice self-awareness and emotional resilience by recognizing and acknowledging your feelings without judgment or criticism.

- Cultivate healthy outlets for expressing emotions, such as journaling, talking to a trusted friend or therapist, or engaging in creative activities like art or music.

- Challenge negative thought patterns and beliefs that contribute to emotional eating, and reframe them with positive affirmations and self-compassion.

Mindful Eating Practices:
- Tune into your body's hunger and fullness cues by practicing mindful eating techniques, such as eating slowly, savoring each bite, and paying attention to the sensory experience of food.

- Pause and check in with yourself before reaching for food, asking yourself if you're truly hungry or if you're eating in response to emotions or stress.

- Create a peaceful eating environment free from distractions, such as television, phones, or computers, to enhance mindfulness and enjoyment of meals.

- Practice portion control by serving yourself smaller portions and avoiding eating directly from containers or packages.

Healthy Coping Strategies:

- Build a toolbox of healthy coping strategies to use in times of stress or emotional distress, such as engaging in hobbies, practicing gratitude, or spending time with loved ones.

- Distract yourself from emotional eating urges by engaging in activities that promote relaxation and enjoyment, such as reading, listening to music, or going for a walk.

- Plan ahead for challenging situations by anticipating potential triggers for emotional eating and developing a plan to cope with them proactively.

By incorporating stress management techniques, emotional regulation strategies, mindful eating practices, and healthy coping strategies into their daily routine, individuals can effectively manage stress and emotional eating to support their weight loss efforts. By cultivating self-awareness, resilience, and healthier habits, individuals can navigate challenging situations with greater ease and achieve long-term success in their weight loss journey.

CHAPTER 8: OVERCOMING PLATEAUS AND SETBACKS

Common reasons for weight loss plateaus and how to break through them.

Weight loss plateaus are a common occurrence in the journey towards achieving a healthier weight. These plateaus can be frustrating, but understanding the reasons behind them and implementing strategies to overcome them can help reignite progress and keep you on track towards your goals. Here are some common reasons for weight loss plateaus and effective ways to break through them.

Metabolic Adaptation:

- *Reason:* Your body may adapt to your reduced calorie intake and increased physical activity levels over time, leading to a slowdown in metabolic rate and weight loss progress.

- *Solution:* Shake up your routine by incorporating high-intensity interval training (HIIT), strength training, or varying your exercise intensity and duration. Additionally, consider cycling your calorie intake by incorporating refeed days or increasing your calorie intake slightly for a short period to reset your metabolism.

Inconsistent Caloric Intake:

- *Reason:* Inadvertently consuming more calories than you realize, whether it's from larger portion sizes, mindless snacking, or underestimating calorie content in foods.

- *Solution:* Track your food intake meticulously using a food diary or calorie-tracking app to ensure accuracy. Pay attention to portion sizes, practice mindful eating, and be aware of hidden sources of calories such as sauces, dressings, and beverages.

Lack of Sleep:

- *Reason:* Inadequate sleep can disrupt hormonal balance, including increased levels of cortisol (the stress hormone) and decreased levels of leptin (the hormone that signals fullness), leading to weight gain and difficulty losing weight.

- *Solution:* Prioritize quality sleep by establishing a consistent sleep schedule, creating a relaxing bedtime routine, and optimizing your sleep environment. Aim for 7-9 hours of sleep per night to support weight loss efforts.

Stress and Emotional Eating:

- *Reason:* Stress can trigger emotional eating and cravings for high-calorie comfort foods, leading to overeating and weight loss plateaus.

- *Solution:* Implement stress management techniques such as mindfulness meditation, deep breathing exercises, yoga, or engaging in hobbies to reduce stress levels. Find healthy coping mechanisms for managing emotions instead of turning to food for comfort.

Underestimating Non-Exercise Activity Thermogenesis (NEAT):

- *Reason:* NEAT encompasses the calories burned through daily activities such as walking, standing, and fidgeting, which can vary significantly among individuals.

- *Solution:* Increase your NEAT by incorporating more movement into your daily routine, such as taking the stairs instead of the elevator, standing while on phone calls, or going for short walks throughout the day.

Water Retention:

- *Reason:* Sodium intake, hormonal fluctuations, and dehydration can all contribute to water retention, masking true fat loss progress on the scale.

- *Solution:* Stay hydrated by drinking plenty of water throughout the day and reducing sodium intake by avoiding processed foods and opting for whole, unprocessed options. Be patient and trust the process, focusing on non-scale victories such as improved energy levels, strength gains, and clothing fit.

Weight loss plateaus are a natural part of the journey towards achieving a healthier weight and can be overcome with patience, persistence, and strategic adjustments. By identifying the underlying reasons for plateaus and implementing targeted strategies to break through them, you can continue making progress towards your weight loss goals and maintain long-term success. Remember to focus on sustainable lifestyle changes, celebrate small victories along the way, and seek support from professionals or peers if needed.

Coping strategies for dealing with setbacks and staying committed to your goals.

Setbacks are an inevitable part of any journey towards achieving goals, including weight loss and overall health improvement. While setbacks can be discouraging, they also present valuable opportunities for learning, growth, and resilience. Here are some effective coping strategies to help you navigate setbacks and stay committed to your goals, empowering you to overcome obstacles and continue moving forward on your journey to wellness.

Practice Self-Compassion:

Recognize that setbacks are a normal and unavoidable part of the process. Instead of being self-critical or judgmental, treat yourself with kindness and understanding.

Remind yourself that setbacks do not define your worth or capabilities. Focus on your progress and accomplishments, no matter how small, and acknowledge the effort you've put in towards your goals.

Reframe Negative Thoughts:

Challenge negative thoughts and beliefs that arise in response to setbacks. Instead of viewing setbacks as failures, reframe them as opportunities for growth, learning, and course correction.

Adopt a growth mindset, recognizing setbacks as temporary obstacles that can be overcome with perseverance, determination, and resilience.

Reflect and Learn:

Take time to reflect on the factors that contributed to the setback, such as external challenges, internal barriers, or unhelpful behaviors. Identify any patterns or triggers that may have led to the setback.

Use setbacks as opportunities for self-reflection and self-awareness. Consider what you can learn from the experience and how you can apply those lessons to improve your approach moving forward.

Set Realistic Expectations:

Adjust your expectations and goals to be realistic, achievable, and sustainable. Avoid setting overly ambitious goals that may set you up for disappointment or burnout.

Break down larger goals into smaller, more manageable milestones. Celebrate progress along the way and recognize that slow progress is still progress.

Seek Support:
Reach out to friends, family members, or support groups for encouragement, empathy, and advice during challenging times. Share your experiences, struggles, and victories with others who understand and can offer support.

Consider working with a coach, therapist, or mentor who can provide guidance, accountability, and personalized strategies for overcoming setbacks and staying on track towards your goals.

Practice Resilience:
Cultivate resilience by developing coping skills and strategies to bounce back from setbacks stronger than before. Draw upon your inner

strength, determination, and resourcefulness to persevere in the face of adversity.

Focus on what you can control and take proactive steps towards positive change, rather than dwelling on past setbacks or things beyond your control.

Stay Focused on Your Why:
Reconnect with your intrinsic motivations and reasons for pursuing your goals. Remind yourself of the benefits and rewards that await you on the other side of setbacks, such as improved health, increased energy, and enhanced well-being.

Visualize your goals, envisioning yourself achieving success and embodying the qualities of resilience, determination, and perseverance that are necessary for reaching them.

Dealing with setbacks is an integral part of any journey towards achieving goals, including weight loss and overall health improvement. By practicing self-compassion, reframing negative thoughts, reflecting and learning from experiences, setting realistic expectations, seeking support, practicing resilience, and staying focused on your intrinsic motivations, you can navigate setbacks with grace and determination, staying committed to your goals and ultimately achieving success. Remember that setbacks are temporary obstacles that can be overcome with perseverance, resilience, and a positive mindset.

CHAPTER 9: MAINTENANCE AND BEYOND

Tips for transitioning from weight loss to weight maintenance.

Transitioning from a period of active weight loss to weight maintenance requires a shift in mindset, habits, and strategies. While the focus shifts from calorie restriction and rapid weight loss to long-term sustainability and balance, it's essential to implement strategies that support weight maintenance while still promoting overall health and well-being. Here are some practical tips to help you successfully transition from weight loss to weight maintenance and sustain your progress for the long term.

Gradually Increase Caloric Intake:
Gradually increase your calorie intake from the reduced levels used during weight loss to a level that supports weight maintenance. This allows your metabolism to adapt slowly and helps prevent rapid weight regain.

Monitor your weight and adjust your calorie intake as needed to find the right balance for weight maintenance without excessive restriction or overeating.

Focus on Nutrient-Dense Foods:
Continue prioritizing nutrient-dense foods such as fruits, vegetables, lean proteins, whole grains, and healthy fats in your diet. These foods provide essential nutrients while helping you feel satisfied and energized.

Be mindful of portion sizes and practice moderation with higher-calorie foods to avoid excessive calorie intake.

Incorporate Regular Physical Activity:

Maintain a consistent exercise routine that includes a combination of cardiovascular exercise, strength training, and flexibility exercises. Aim for at least 150 minutes of moderate-intensity aerobic activity or 75 minutes of vigorous-intensity activity per week, along with muscle-strengthening activities on two or more days per week.

Find activities you enjoy and make them a regular part of your routine to help you stay active and support weight maintenance.

Practice Mindful Eating:

Continue practicing mindful eating techniques, such as paying attention to hunger and fullness cues, eating slowly, and savoring each bite. This can help prevent overeating and promote a healthier relationship with food.

Be mindful of emotional eating triggers and find alternative coping mechanisms to manage stress, boredom, or other emotions without turning to food.

Monitor Your Progress:

Regularly monitor your weight and body measurements to track your progress and detect any changes early on. This can help you identify patterns, adjust your behaviors as needed, and prevent significant weight regain.

Keep a food diary or use a tracking app to monitor your food intake and ensure you're staying within your calorie goals for weight maintenance.

Establish Healthy Habits:

Focus on establishing healthy lifestyle habits that support long-term weight maintenance, such as getting adequate sleep, managing stress effectively, staying hydrated, and practicing self-care.

Surround yourself with a supportive environment that encourages healthy behaviors and reinforces your commitment to maintaining your weight loss achievements.

Be Flexible and Adaptive:
Be prepared for fluctuations in weight and recognize that weight maintenance is not always linear. Allow yourself flexibility and adaptability in your approach, and be willing to make adjustments as needed based on your individual needs and circumstances.

Remember that achieving and maintaining a healthy weight is a lifelong journey, and it's normal to encounter challenges along the way. Stay patient, resilient, and committed to your goals, and celebrate your successes, no matter how small.

Transitioning from weight loss to weight maintenance requires a shift in mindset, habits, and strategies. By gradually increasing calorie intake, focusing on nutrient-dense foods, incorporating regular physical activity, practicing mindful eating, monitoring progress, establishing healthy habits, and being flexible and adaptive, you can successfully maintain your weight loss achievements for the long term. Remember that weight maintenance is a lifelong journey, and staying committed to healthy behaviors and habits is key to sustaining your progress and enjoying lasting health and well-being.

Importance of adopting lifelong habits for overall health and well-being.

In the pursuit of optimal health and well-being, adopting lifelong habits that promote physical, mental, and emotional wellness is essential. While short-term changes can yield temporary benefits, it is the sustained commitment to healthy habits over time that leads to lasting improvements in quality of life. Here are the importance of adopting lifelong habits for overall health and well-being and how these habits contribute to a fulfilling and vibrant life.

Sustainable Health Outcomes:

Lifelong habits provide the foundation for sustainable health outcomes that extend beyond short-term fixes or temporary solutions. By integrating healthy behaviors into daily life, individuals can achieve lasting improvements in physical fitness, weight management, and chronic disease prevention.

Prevention of Chronic Diseases:

Lifelong habits such as regular physical activity, balanced nutrition, stress management, and adequate sleep play a crucial role in preventing chronic diseases such as heart disease, diabetes, obesity, and certain cancers.

Consistent adherence to healthy habits can help reduce risk factors associated with chronic diseases, improve overall health markers, and enhance longevity and quality of life.

Mental and Emotional Well-being:

Adopting lifelong habits that prioritize mental and emotional well-being, such as mindfulness, relaxation techniques, positive self-talk, and social connection, contributes to greater resilience, emotional balance, and psychological health.

These habits promote stress reduction, enhance coping skills, and foster a sense of fulfillment, purpose, and connection in life.

Long-Term Weight Management:

Sustainable weight management requires lifelong habits that support healthy eating, regular physical activity, portion control, and mindful eating practices.

By incorporating these habits into daily life, individuals can achieve and maintain a healthy weight without resorting to fad diets, extreme measures, or yo-yo dieting cycles.

Improved Quality of Life:
Lifelong habits contribute to an improved quality of life by enhancing physical vitality, mental clarity, emotional resilience, and overall well-being.

By prioritizing self-care, balance, and holistic health, individuals can enjoy greater energy levels, productivity, creativity, and fulfillment in all areas of life.

Role Modeling for Others:
Adopting lifelong habits sets a positive example for others, including family members, friends, and communities, inspiring them to prioritize their health and well-being.

By demonstrating the benefits of healthy living through actions and behaviors, individuals can empower others to make positive changes and create a ripple effect of wellness within their social circles and beyond.

Long-Term Sustainability:

Lifelong habits are sustainable habits that can be maintained over the long term, regardless of life's challenges, transitions, or obstacles.

By cultivating resilience, adaptability, and a growth mindset, individuals can navigate through life's ups and downs while staying committed to their health and well-being goals.

Adopting lifelong habits for overall health and well-being is essential for achieving sustained improvements in physical, mental, and emotional wellness. By prioritizing sustainable health outcomes, preventing chronic diseases, nurturing mental and emotional well-being, managing weight effectively, enhancing quality of life, role modeling for others, and embracing long-term sustainability, individuals can cultivate a lifestyle that promotes vitality, resilience, and fulfillment. Remember that small, consistent changes over time lead to significant and lasting results, and the journey towards lifelong health and well-being is an ongoing process of growth, discovery, and self-care.

CONCLUSION

In concluding "The Most Proven and Effective Way to Achieve Weight Loss" it's imperative to reflect on the journey embarked upon, the lessons learned, and the transformations experienced. Throughout this book, we've delved into the multifaceted approach required to achieve sustainable weight loss effectively, emphasizing the importance of adopting a holistic and balanced approach to health and well-being.

We've explored the fundamental principles of weight loss, including creating a calorie deficit, understanding metabolism, and the significance of the mind-body connection in shaping our eating habits and behaviors. By embracing healthy eating habits, regular physical activity, and mindful practices, readers have gained insight into how to achieve and maintain a healthy weight while prioritizing their overall health and wellness.

Moreover, we've addressed common challenges and setbacks encountered along the weight loss journey, providing practical strategies for overcoming obstacles with resilience, patience, and determination. By reframing setbacks as opportunities for growth and learning, readers are empowered to navigate through challenges with grace and fortitude, staying committed to their goals despite the inevitable ups and downs.

As readers transition from weight loss to weight maintenance, they're encouraged to embrace lifelong habits that support their health and well-being, recognizing that sustainable changes lead to lasting results. By prioritizing self-care, balance, and holistic wellness, individuals can cultivate a lifestyle that promotes vitality, resilience, and fulfillment.

In essence, "The Most Proven and Effective Way to Achieve Weight Loss" is not just about shedding pounds—it's about reclaiming control of our health, nurturing our bodies, and embracing a positive relationship with food, exercise, and self-care. It's about recognizing that true transformation comes from within, and that by honoring our bodies and minds, we can unlock our full potential and live a life of abundance and vitality.

As readers close the pages of this book, may they carry with them the knowledge, inspiration, and empowerment to continue their journey towards better health and well-being, one step at a time. Remember, the path to weight loss and wellness is unique to each individual, but with dedication, perseverance, and a commitment to self-care, anything is possible.

Here's to your health, happiness, and lifelong well-being.